CARBOHYDRATE CONTROLLED DIET

A Balanced Carb Blood Sugar Solution To
Diabetes Management (CCD Diet)

BY MATHEA FORD, RD/LD, MBA

INTRODUCTION AND DISCLAIMER

<u>Why I wrote this book</u> - In my book, I wrote extensively about how to take your diabetes diet to the next level and get it under control. I want to make sure you are able to do this yourself, and give you actionable tips to use.

What I have found through the emails and requests of my readers is that it is difficult to find information about a healthy and reasonable diabetes diet that is actionable. I want you to know that is what I intend to provide in all my books. Especially this one. You can take these recipes and create several weeks of meals that you and your family will enjoy and they all fit a person with diabetes and their needs.

I wrote this book with you in mind: the person with diabetes who does not know where to start or can't seem to get the answers that you need from other sources. This book will provide help that is applicable to your diabetes diet – no matter if it's type 1 or 2 or pre-diabetes.

Who am I? I am a registered dietitian in the USA who has been working with people with diabetes for my entire 17 + years of experience. I have a website that provides diabetes meal plans for all stages of diabetes – check it out at
http://www.healthydietmenusforyou.com/

Find all my books on amazon on my author page:
http://www.amazon.com/Mathea-Ford/e/B008E1E7IS/

<u>My goals are simple</u> – to give some answers and to create an understanding of what is typical. It will not necessarily be what happens in your case, as everyone is an individual. I may simplify things in an effort to write them so that I feel you can learn the most from the information. This may mean that I don't say the exact things that your doctor would say. If you don't understand, please ask your doctor.

I want you to know, I am not a medical doctor and I am not aware of your particular condition. Information in this book is current as of publication, but may or may not have changed. This book is not meant to substitute for medical treatment for you, your friends, your caregivers, or your family members. You should not base treatment decisions solely on what is contained in this book. Develop your treatment plan with your doctors, nurses and the other medical professionals on your team.

In other words, I am not responsible for your medical care. I am providing this book for information and entertainment purposes, not medical diagnoses. Please consult with your doctor about any questions that you have about your particular case.

TABLE OF CONTENTS

Introduction...7

What is Diabetes? 13

What is a Carbohydrate Controlled Diet?........................23

Benefits of a Carbohydrate Controlled Diet 31

Getting Motivated 37

How to Follow the Diet...43

Carbohydrate Counting and Label Reading 49

Quick Steps to Greater Carbohydrate Control................59

Carbohydrate Counting Plan..67

The First Week...79

Correcting Mistakes...83

Recipes 89

Summary and Next Steps..101

Worksheets:..103

Other Titles By Mathea Ford 105

INTRODUCTION

THE PURPOSE OF THIS BOOK

Your health is important. It makes sense to eat a well-balanced and thought-conscious set of meals each day, but many of us do precisely the opposite. We eat on the run and without thinking. Life is so fast paced that it is difficult to plan ahead and for many people, nutrition can be sadly lacking. We live off of heavily processed foods that have little in terms of nutritional value and are filled with substances to promote the shelf-life of these products. Carefully concealed within processed foods are flavor additives. Products are often overloaded with unnecessary sugars and salts. It's no wonder many of us feel less than energized or simply unwell.

Adopting a carbohydrate controlled diet is a positive decision for everyone and in particular, for those with diabetes. You may find the calculations process a little confusing in the beginning. It is all about understanding nutritional values and comprehending how food affects you. Once you learn to understand and control the amount of carbohydrates that are consumed each day, your health will become much more stable as a result. This is especially important for people with diabetes as the nature of the disease makes it difficult to control your blood sugar levels on a day to day basis.

Understanding the food that you eat and learning to embrace the idea that you are responsible for your own health is an informed choice. The carbohydrate controlled diet is not about eliminating carbohydrates, but about understanding their relevance. A carbohydrate controlled diet is a meal plan where you plan out the amount of carbohydrate at each meal so it is divided up throughout the day. This keeps you from overeating at any part of the day and at your meals.

The key to embarking upon this type of eating means consuming foods that contain equal amounts of carbohydrate and nutrient rich-foods throughout the day, and at each meal. It's all about consistency and balance with what you eat. This enables your body to avoid having to endure those extreme highs and lows as blood sugar levels fluctuate. Balance means a healthier way of life, more energy, clarity of mind and the ability to simply enjoy life more.

A carbohydrate controlled diet differs from other types of diets because it is adapted to the individual, and it becomes more 'a way of life' than a diet per se. It allows you to gain a greater insight into the needs of your own body and to work towards greater health and well-being by taking care of the nutritional requirements you have without overdoing the carbohydrates and sugars.

There are sections within this book on portion size and a list of carbohydrates that will provide you with an excellent starting point. This book looks at how to prepare your mindset for the changes, so that you fully understand the foundations of this lifestyle change. It's all about adapting and finding a process that suits your body. Although calories are an important factor, the requirements differ for each individual and the amount of exercise each day has to be taken into consideration when trying to determine a precise meal plan.

The more practiced you become, the easier it is to establish healthy and balanced meals that contain equal portions of carbohydrates balanced with fat and protein. This calculated approach to food ensures that your blood sugar levels remain stable with little variation in blood sugar after eating. It's a healthy approach and there is no need to feel deprived because sustenance from all of the main food groups should be included. This ensures that all of the relevant vitamins and minerals are absorbed into your body avoiding any deficiencies. This doesn't cure diabetes, but it can make it far more manageable. Bottom line: You are going to eat a balanced amount of the different nutrients instead of unbalanced meals with too much sugar or carbohydrate.

LEARNING TO CHANGE YOUR DIETARY HABITS
When you have become accustomed to eating certain food types or eating on the run for a long period of time, it can be difficult to

revamp your approach. If your life is busy, then your main concern will be finding time to organize and to prepare a healthier menu for the week. This additional time spent on preparation, however, is important and can make a big difference to your overall health in the short term. It's all about changing your mindset, deciding to embrace the changes and evaluating the results after a few weeks. Start with knowing you can complete this challenge, and all it requires is some forethought and preparation.

Diabetes is a serious condition regardless of which type of diabetes that you have. It has long-term health consequences as well as short-term negative influences. When you consider making changes on a practical level, it is worth embracing the concepts of the carbohydrate controlled diet which is tasty, nutritious and can make a huge positive impact on your health.

If you have a family to cater for, there is no need to be concerned with providing different food types as the carbohydrate controlled diet is safe and nutritious for all.

COMPREHENDING THE IMPORTANCE OF A CARBOHYDRATE CONTROLLED MEAL PLAN

Making these changes to your dietary lifestyle isn't about your embracing some fad diet which promises substantial health claims including the potential to lose weight overnight. It is about making an important choice to care for your body by feeding it the right nutrients required to ensure that your body remains consistently energized and refreshed.

Weight loss certainly is achievable on this diet but this is a positive by-product. This is important for all and not simply for those suffering with diabetes. There will be an improvement to triglycerides and HDL levels, improved blood cholesterol levels, and lower blood pressure for all those who successfully start and continue to monitor the quantities of carbohydrates each day, simply through better choices of food and better blood sugar control.

Carbohydrates should not be avoided. Nor should they be deemed bad for the body. In fact, your body instinctively prefers the energy that it gains from carbohydrates. It is, as previously stated, about balancing the intake. With diabetes, it is so important to establish an eating plan that really works for you. This means portion control with an emphasis on the quantity of carbohydrates at each mealtime. This way you will be able to avoid those fluctuating sugar levels and the greater risk of more serious complications in the future.

Balancing carbohydrates with insulin requirements can be difficult but it is important that the individual take an intuitive approach to their health. Gradually, with trial and error, your body will tell you what works and what does not as you are more able to sense how it reacts to blood sugar changes. Discuss any changes to a prescription for diabetes or related condition with your doctor prior to implementation.

WHAT IS DIABETES?

DIABETES TYPES

If you have diabetes, you will know just how overwhelming and life-changing it can be. It is a disease that affects how your body uses blood glucose - commonly known as blood sugar. Glucose provides the fuel for your brain as well as for your body and it is vital for your health. While there are different types of diabetes, having the condition simply means that you have too great an amount of glucose in your blood and it has to be managed. The reasons for the increase in glucose will vary depending on the type of diabetes and the cause should always be determined while managing the risks. Nonetheless, once you have been diagnosed with diabetes, your eating habits will change.

As your body breaks down the carbohydrate that you eat, it turns to glucose in your digestive system. Then it is absorbed into your bloodstream and as glucose levels increase, your body responds by releasing insulin. Insulin is a hormone secreted from within the pancreas. This compound is vital for everyday health and well-being as your body uses glucose to generate energy used for healing, growth, and movement. To be able to utilize this fuel, the glucose has to be moved to the cells from the bloodstream. For this to happen, it needs insulin. When the pancreas works sufficiently, the right levels of insulin are made allowing glucose to be absorbed.

How Insulin Works

Glucose is a source of energy from carbohydrates and is produced from the food that you eat. Glucose (blood sugar) is absorbed into the blood stream and is helped into the cells by insulin.

Insulin is a hormone which is produced in the gland called the pancreas and it acts as a key allowing glucose to access the cells. Glucose is then used to produce energy, and the process is as follows:

1. Insulin enters the bloodstream from the pancreas

2. As the insulin circulates, this enables sugar (glucose) to enter the cells

3. Insulin lowers the level of sugar within the bloodstream by letting the glucose into the cells

4. When the glucose level has dropped, the pancreas stops secreting insulin.

Excess amounts of insulin cause the body to store extra blood sugar (glucose) as fat, causing weight gain. Insulin easily converts glucose to fatty tissue in the body.

Type 1 Diabetes

Your immune system actually starts to turn inwards, to attack, and to ultimately destroy the cells within your pancreas. If insufficient levels of insulin are created naturally within the pancreas, you can feel tired or weak and this is because your cells are unable to access glucose. In the case of Type 1 diabetes, you are required to replace your body's insulin because it no longer makes the insulin you need. Type 1 diabetes often occurs as a result of an infection or an injury to the pancreas, although not all causes are known. Type 1 Diabetes can occur at any age, although it is more typically diagnosed during childhood or adolescence.

SYMPTOMS
The symptoms for Type 1 Diabetes can occur very suddenly and include:

Fatigue

Blurred Vision

Weight-Loss

Frequent Urination

An Increased Thirst

PRE-DIABETES
It is always worth having regular blood glucose levels checks even if there is no current confirmation of diabetes. You may still be at risk. Those who develop type 2 diabetes may have

experienced a period of time known as pre-diabetes and where there are elevated blood glucose levels, but they may not be high enough to actually receive official diagnosis. It is often referred to as IGT or impaired glucose tolerance/impaired fasting glucose -IFG. When you have this condition, it is important to keep your blood sugars within normal range to keep it from progressing to full-blown diabetes. You are also at risk and should have regular checks if you had gestational diabetes during your pregnancy.

SYMPTOMS

Because many people have pre-diabetes and are not even aware of it, it is a good idea to be able to identify changes within the body as it is still possible at this point to prevent the actual onset of diabetes type 2, simply by making substantial changes to the diet. There are no clear signs and symptoms, but of those experienced, they may mirror those of type 2 diabetes. The main thing is to have your primary care doctor check your blood sugar every year as part of your checkup.

TYPE 2 DIABETES

Type 2 diabetes is another type of diabetes and it affects the ability to use glucose even though you still make insulin. It is different from type 1 in that either your body resists the insulin effects, or it just does not produce enough insulin so as to maintain normal glucose levels. Type 2 diabetes typically affects adults more commonly, but it affects children too. The condition can be managed fairly well by regulating the diet, exercising and by ensuring a healthy weight is maintained. It may seem relatively easy to ignore type 2 diabetes in the early stages, but left unchecked it can become dangerous. This is because diabetes can affect the function of your heart, eyes, kidneys, nerves, and blood vessels. Complications may develop slowly, but they can become life-threatening and should be treated accordingly. Approximately 26 million Americans have diabetes, or about 8% of the U.S. Population according to the CDC.

SYMPTOMS
Because type 2 diabetes can develop slowly and over a period of time, it is important to check for the symptoms and to seek medical advice if any of the symptoms sound familiar:

Increased Thirst

More Frequent Urination

Weight –Loss / Weight Gain

Increased Hunger

Fatigue

Blurred Vision

Slow Healing Sores

Darker Areas of Skin in Creases (neck and armpits).

Type 2 Diabetes is a serious condition. It is not fully understood why some people develop this disease but it is known that there are certain risks that can increase the potential to contract diabetes. It is becoming far more common across the globe and people's dietary choices are relevant to their risk, as well as many other lifestyle choices.

Activity: The less active you are the higher your risk

Being Overweight: If you are overweight, then this is a primary risk. In fact, the greater the amount of fatty tissue, the more likely your cells will become resistant to insulin. Additionally, if the fat is stored mainly on the abdomen, then the risk increases.

Family History: If there is a history of type 2 diabetes in the family, then the risk is greater.

Race: Research has not yet revealed why but certain races such as Blacks, American Indians, Asian Indians and Hispanics are more prone to developing the disease than others.

Age: The risk also increases after the age of 45.

TREATMENTS FOR DIABETES

There is no known cure for diabetes and prescribed treatments will vary but once diagnosis takes place, the person will have many changes to their daily life. It's vital that blood sugar levels (glucose) are kept stable and as close to normal as possible. Much of the treatment can be self-managed including:

Healthy Eating

Exercising Regularly

Monitoring Blood Sugar

Diabetes Medicine – as prescribed by your doctor

When you monitor your glucose levels, your doctor will suggest regular checks. This is because it is only by frequent checks that levels can be determined to ensure that they are within the safe zone. Diabetes affects people on an individual level. For some there will be some foods that may cause a spike in the sugar levels while for others, they do not have the same response. Usually, in time, the person with diabetes can tell when their levels are unstable, but some people remain dangerously high consistently.

FACTORS AFFECTING YOUR BLOOD SUGAR LEVELS

Food: This will certainly affect your sugar levels and over a period of time you will begin to know all of the foods that have the potential to raise blood sugar levels. This book focuses on carbohydrates and how to control them which in turn leads to keeping you feeling more balanced once those sugar levels stabilize. Keeping a food journal enables you to be more aware of triggers that can make your levels remain too high by eating too many servings of carbohydrate. Your blood sugars are usually higher one to two hours following your meal as your body releases insulin and works to bring it down.

Medication: Any medication may affect your sugar levels and if this happens, treatment may need to be changed. Talking to your doctor about changes is very important prior to making any adjustments. Be informed about the potential of a medication to cause low blood sugars and how to respond to the event.

Illness: When you become ill, your body will sometimes produce hormones that could upset the balance of sugar levels, and cause them to be elevated even without any intake of carbohydrate.

Stress: Rising or fluctuating stress levels can also affect your hormones and this can play havoc with your insulin levels. When you face stressful situations, adrenaline is released from the adrenal glands preparing your body for what is known as the 'fight or flight' syndrome. As adrenalin rushes into your body, both your breathing and heart rate increase and your senses become more finely tuned. Nutrients are also released to prepare for muscular activity, and blood flow to less important organs decreases. Your body stays in this heightened state of alertness until danger has passed and the threat has been eradicated.

These changes happen instinctively when faced with dangerous situations, but they also happen when you face difficult situations in everyday life. You might not be facing life-threatening events but your body still responds as if threatened. Your body reacts as if it feels under pressure and your body remains continuously in a state of fight or flight until the stress is gone. This has an incredibly negative impact on your body as you overwork your heart, but you also impact your digestive system and the immune system.

Alcohol: When you drink alcohol, you can very easily disrupt your blood sugar levels so it's important to watch the quantities of alcohol that are consumed. Avoid drinking too much on a frequent basis. Alcohol can decrease your inhibitions and your appetite, causing you to eat more as well as to consume less healthy options. Some medications may be negatively affected by alcohol consumption.

Hormonal Fluctuations: Women's hormone levels fluctuate throughout the month as their menstrual cycle progresses, and in the week prior to a period, blood sugar levels can rise and dip. Similarly, menopause can trigger the same response, possibly even more erratically as the body manages changing hormone levels. Over time you can track your blood glucose levels to see if they change based on hormone levels.

Physical Fitness: Exercise can be really beneficial for everyone including those with diabetes. Type 2 diabetes sufferers respond well to increased exercise and to a healthy diet. For many people, a healthy lifestyle staves off the need for medicine or at least reduces the potential for health to decrease. It doesn't matter how fit the individual is, even a little exercise can make a difference and provides many benefits. Ideally, you should exercise for approximately 150 minutes per week. Exercise should be spread out over the week for maximum benefit. This will be an important part of the carbohydrate controlled diet. It is important to start off slowly and to build up a regular exercise program as fitness increases.

WHAT IS A CARBOHYDRATE CONTROLLED DIET?

OVERVIEW

Anyone interested in increasing their health and well-being can begin a carbohydrate controlled diet as it provides positive dietary changes for the whole family. For people with diabetes especially, these changes are important as they serve to maintain consistent blood sugar levels. The concept may appear a little complicated initially, but it simply means increasing your knowledge of food and nutrition and planning the foods that you eat. Make sure you have all of the regular nutrients while ensuring a stable and consistent quantity of carbohydrates throughout the day, each and every day. The benefits of doing so start to become apparent quickly.

The first thing that you need to consider is that each meal will consist of 50%-60% carbohydrates. You should choose whole grain, low-medium glycemic index, and less processed carbohydrates that are absorbed slowly and eat your meals at approximately the same times each day when possible. To make it easier to comprehend – all carbohydrates once digested are broken down into glucose; it is the journey to this state that determines whether they are deemed healthy or not. The whole grains and less processed carbohydrates are healthier because they retain many of the healthy vitamins and minerals, as well as additional fiber your body needs.

If you eat too many carbohydrates as a portion of your diet, it can be dangerous. Your diet certainly has a direct bearing on your brain health. High levels of carbohydrates and eventually blood sugars can cause problems with your memory, language and even your judgment. This also adds weight to the fact that consistent levels of carbohydrates is the way forward and so are good for your mental capabilities as well as for your energy levels. If you eat a balanced diet with a consistent level of carbohydrates (that are healthy – whole grain, low-medium glycemic index, and less processed), you will more likely have healthy blood sugar levels.

FEATURES

Nutrition and the debate over carbohydrates can be confusing in the best of times. But the great thing about a carbohydrate controlled diet is that it is easier to plan regular meals once you understand the concept. It is simply an acquired state of mind and understanding as to why you choose specific carbohydrates (good vs. bad carbohydrates) and the quantities that are required (number of portions). Additionally, you need to establish regular meal times each day.

First, it is important to understand that foods contain valuable nutrients and energy. But there are two typical forms of carbohydrates which are:

- Sugars including fructose, lactose and glucose.

- Starches including rice, breads, grains, cereals and starchy vegetables such as corn or potatoes.

Carbohydrates are broken down into glucose by the body and then absorbed into the bloodstream through the digestive tract. The glucose (blood sugar) travels into the cells using insulin and this is where it is converted into energy.

As you can imagine, keeping your body's glucose levels stable is important because it maintains your energy levels and enables you to carry out your daily duties. You have to watch what you eat and more importantly, keep track of all of the carbohydrates consumed, and watch your portions carefully. What matters is the type of carbohydrate eaten.

Opting for whole grain foods or fruit is a much healthier option than eating a plate of French fries every day. Whole grains are healthier because your body takes longer to break them down and absorb them. This allows time for your body's insulin to respond more evenly. You don't have the huge spikes in blood sugar but instead a steady rise and fall of blood sugar levels that is closer to a normal response. This is the educational part of understanding carbohydrates and once you can identify those that are healthier, you can adapt your diet accordingly, avoiding those peaks and valleys of glucose spikes that derail your progress and make you feel tired and mentally exhausted.

GUIDELINES

Once you learn all about the different carbohydrates, it will be simpler to devise a set meal plan. On a carbohydrate controlled diet, you need to typically eat between 50%- 60% of carbohydrates at each meal. This may be a mixture of good and bad carbohydrates with the emphasis on good carbohydrates of course. Portion control is important. But it is not as simple at this. It is about the nutrients within your food choices too. Are you getting sufficient vitamins and minerals? Are you eating too high a saturated fat content? Do you have too much sugar in your diet? You need to balance your food intake but consider your nutritional needs too. It is worth emphasizing that there are variables which will affect the quantity of carbohydrates per meal. You need to consider your age, height, build, whether you are trying to lose weight, how much you exercise and any medication that you are on.

In general, many people have an idea of how many calories they should eat to lose weight. If you don't, you can use the following information to determine your calorie needs.

Women: Weight in pounds X 11 (example: 120 pound woman X 11 = 1320 baseline calories)

Men: Weight in pounds X 12 (example 200 pound man X 12 = 2400 baseline calories)

Then you multiply by the factor for your activity level –

1.2 = sitting all day

1.3 = exercise 1-2 days per week, somewhat active

1.4 = exercise 2-3 days per week

1.5 = exercise more than 3 times per week, active

1.7 = exercise hard daily, very active

For the woman – 1320 calories X 1.2 (sitting all day) = 1584 calories

For the man – 2400 calories X 1.2 (sitting all day) = 2880 calories

This indicates how many calories you burn in a day. In order to lose weight, you should reduce the calories by about 10 – 15 %. This will give you a calorie deficit and allow your body to burn some of the stored fat for energy. Your body will burn fat for energy more readily when the carbohydrate you provide is not simple sugars and high fructose corn syrup. In other words, your body will treat donut calories different from whole wheat bread with peanut butter. It will take time to absorb the bread and not turn the glucose into stored fat like it will for the donut.

At this point, you will need to figure out how many calories and grams of carbohydrate that you should eat. Carbohydrates should consist of about 50% of your calories – so if you were to take the above examples – I will do the calculations for you:

Woman – 1584 calories X 0.50 = 792 calories. So, 792 calories each day should come from carbohydrates. How many grams of carbohydrates does that equal? 792 / 4 (4 calories in a gram of carbohydrate) = 198 gm of carbohydrate per day. You can divide that out as 45 gm of carbohydrate per meal (3 servings at 15 gm each) + 2 snacks with 30 gm carbohydrate each.

Man – 2880 calories X 0.50 = 1440 calories. So 1440 calories in the day should come from carbohydrates. In this case, how many grams should be in carbohydrates for the day? 1440 calories / 4 (4 calories in a gram of carbohydrate) = 360 calories per day. In this case, you can divide that up into 3 meals with 75 grams each (5 servings). And then you have 9 servings of carbohydrates left – basically 2 snacks – one with 4 carbohydrate servings and one with 5 carbohydrate servings.

WHY SHOULD SOMEONE FOLLOW A CARBOHYDRATE CONTROLLED DIET?

There are far too many fad diets promoted these days and these can be more harmful than good, creating yo-yo dieting syndromes and an irregular weight cycle. This can be especially dangerous for those with health conditions such as diabetes. With careful control of carbohydrate intake, there will be a noticeable reduction of hunger pangs too, leading to easily following the meal plan. People often struggle with their weight because they do not understand the food that they consume, so a healthier eating plan focusing on the quantity of carbohydrates is a good place to start. Controlling carbohydrates does not specifically make you lose weight but, it does increase your energy which means you can get out there and exercise too. A carbohydrate-controlled diet enables the intake to be set at a specific value in this case: 50%-60%. If you consult with a dietitian and they recommend more or less carbohydrate, you should follow their instructions.

BENEFITS OF A CARBOHYDRATE CONTROLLED DIET

WEIGHT LOSS

When you start your journey towards consistent health and begin the carbohydrate controlled diet, it is possible to lose weight fairly naturally. Carbohydrates convert to energy and so it is important to increase the amount of exercise undertaken which enables you to get fitter and healthier more quickly. Monitoring the carbs that you consume is the most important aspect, as is having the right mix of carbohydrates which help to maintain blood sugar levels and to keep diabetes under control. Equally, if there is no diabetes present, it can also work in a preventable way - especially important for those with pre-diabetes or who are at risk. Pre-diabetes can be a danger because you continue to eat foods that are not helping your body to stay healthy and diabetes can develop without warning. Combining the carbohydrates and switching from white rice or white bread to brown rice and whole-wheat products, and utilizing these with other carbohydrates such as beans will help you to eat approximately 50% of carbohydrates with every meal.

Carbohydrates that are high in resistant starch can actually help to speed up your metabolism which is of real benefit if you are trying to lose a little bit of weight. Resistant starch releases fatty acids that actually encourage fat burning as it moves through the digestive system.

Resistant starch is considered the third type of dietary fiber and includes starch and starch degradation content that is not digested in the small intestine. It delivers some of the benefits of those soluble fibers and insoluble fibers and passes through to the large intestine. By comparison, other starches and sugars are turned into glucose easily and are used for short-term energy requirements or become stored.

Resistant starch is much like fiber in your diet, and eating foods that are high in fiber help you get more resistant starch. Eating more fiber is a natural part of a CCD diet because you are eating more unprocessed and whole grains which are higher in fiber. Some examples of foods high in resistant starch include bananas, oatmeal, white beans, lentils, and barley.

REDUCED BLOOD GLUCOSE

With diabetes, making regular checks on blood sugar levels is essential but, with a carbohydrate controlled diet, it is possible to lower blood glucose levels substantially and to maintain this level. It's a productive self-help tool. This reduction of the peaks and valleys of sugar levels is achieved by careful plate portion control and eating regularly throughout the day, the same times each and every day for maximum benefits.

As a person with diabetes, this program will help you keep blood sugar levels near normal which is very healthy.

REDUCING TRIGLYCERIDES
It's important that you understand the effect that triglycerides have on the body. They are a type of fat which is used by your body for energy and while this sounds fairly harmless, if you have high triglycerides then it can raise the risk of heart disease. If you have a blood test for the measurement of cholesterol levels, it will also measure the triglycerides. When your blood sugar level is high, your triglyceride level will be high. The amount of simple sugar and alcohol that you consume significantly affects your blood triglyceride levels.

High triglycerides are typically caused by conditions including:

- Diabetes

- Underactive Thyroid

- Eating more calories than is required/high amounts of sugar

- Drinking excess alcohol

- Kidney Disease

Insulin sensitivity is how strongly you react to the effects of insulin in your body. Many diabetics have decrease insulin sensitivity, causing them to need more insulin over time. It is important to improve insulin sensitivity. If you are insulin sensitive, you will require lower amounts of insulin to lower your blood glucose levels. The levels of insulin sensitivity will vary from person to person and there are tests that can determine your personal level of insulin sensitivity.

For those with diabetes and with low insulin insensitivity, the individual will need larger amounts of insulin. This is released from the pancreas or through insulin injections to keep the blood glucose levels stable. Insulin resistance is an indicator that your body has problems converting glucose and it is important to realize that this can also highlight future potential problems by way of increased cholesterol levels and high blood pressure.

When you follow a carbohydrate controlled diet, your body is able to respond to glucose evenly because glucose is absorbed at a slower rate instead of rushing into the blood stream. This allows even those with low insulin sensitivity to keep blood sugar under control.

When you eat simple sugars they are very easily absorbed into the bloodstream. Because they are almost already broken down to the level your body absorbs them as, they are quickly processed and moved into your bloodstream, raising your blood sugar level in minutes.

However, if you eat complex carbohydrates and whole grains, the body has to break them down further – penetrating the crust or coating of the grain and the n breaking down the complex molecules in to glucose. All this work takes time and causes them to be absorbed at a slower rate. This is why when you need to raise your blood sugar quickly, you drink something like juice. Juice is very easy to absorb and raises blood sugar in a hurry. Of course, that should be followed with a more complex carbohydrate to allow the blood sugar to continue to return to a normal level over time instead of remaining high by eating more sugary foods.

WHY IS INSULIN SENSITIVITY IS IMPORTANT?

If you have low insulin sensitivity, your body can try to over compensate by producing more insulin. High levels of circulating insulin are associated with obesity, heart disease, osteoporosis, high blood pressure, and cancer. If your life is particularly stressful, it is important to manage the stress levels because this can cause reduced insulin sensitivity.

GETTING MOTIVATED

WHEN SHOULD SOMEONE START THIS DIET?

Whether you have type 2 diabetes, pre-diabetes, or simply have concerns about your energy levels and the types of food that you are eating regularly, then don't delay. You instinctively know if your health feels subpar and whether your diabetes is becoming out of control. Once you have read each chapter you will understand how to ascertain the foods to eat and can start to work out a meal plan. You don't need to make radical changes, but simple ones may be the best option for you so that within a week or two, you have incorporated the diet within everyday life. Make the decision to introduce a healthier way of eating and make notes as you work through this book so that you can identify any necessary changes to your normal shopping list.

Initially, it means buying healthier carbohydrates such as brown rice and whole-grain breads (there is more information in later chapters) and choosing a healthier and wide-ranging set of ingredients that provide you with all of the nutrients you need. Once you implement the changes, you will start to feel the benefits in a matter of days.

IDENTIFYING PERSONAL GOALS

Every person has his or her own specific health goals. For many of us, it is to regain energy levels and to feel healthy, alive, and filled with vitality. Remember how you felt when you were young and before you ate food that had been prepared for convenience instead of for nutrients? For those with diabetes, there are greater health issues, because it is important to not let the condition worsen. Identifying individual needs are important because these can become a solid starting point for progression. Everyone has a responsibility to their own health and sometimes it is as simple as sitting down and working out an action plan. Prioritize the list of your requirements – those goals that can be achieved quickly (short term – 1 to 2 weeks), and then the mid-term (2 to 3 months), and finally, the long-term goals (6 months to 1 year). When working out what you need to achieve, think about your health and any areas of concern. This will help you to write a personalized list that will give you something on which to focus.

Some ideas of personal goals might be:

- Eat consistent portion meals 3 times per day and document what I eat

- Take blood sugar levels 3 times per day and meet goal of 120 mg/dL before meals

- Write out a meal plan for the week and use with grocery shopping

KEEPING A LIST OF HEALTH BENEFITS

There are numerous health benefits when embarking on a carbohydrate controlled diet. For many people, the prospect of feeling better with much more energy is very appealing. Many of us are used to living the highs and lows of fluctuating glucose levels and we respond by eating foods that could cause a spike in our glucose levels followed by an unhealthy drop which in turn, leads to even more fluctuations. Think about the times when you suddenly reach for a bar of chocolate because your energy levels plummeted. Getting your glucose levels stable throughout the day will provide you with additional energy for life. It will strip away feelings of tiredness or the unexpected symptoms of diabetes, and life will feel good again. As you embark upon this lifestyle change, you will start to feel better, more energized, and less tired, and it is worth making a note of the improvements as this will help to spur you on.

Try writing down your energy levels daily and see how they change on the diet. Another health benefit is better blood sugar control which leads to fewer complications from diabetes. When you have better blood sugar control, you are less likely to develop eye, nerve, and kidney problems. Write out your blood sugar level goals and track them. Adjust your amount of carbohydrate to meet the goals and observe how you feel. While the long term benefits are great, it helps to see daily progress.

SUPPORT

Changing your diet to one that is going to promote inner health and well-being is a crucial step if you wish to extend your life and to enjoy feeling and looking great. But, as with any life-changing plan, it's good to have a solid support network around you. This is because there will be times when your dedication to the cause dips a little. You will no doubt feel tempted to just snack sometimes or to reach for the wrong food types because you feel a little stressed or tired and feel the need for something that is quick and easy. When others know that you are trying to stick to the carbohydrate controlled diet, it's harder to cheat, and they can help you by not offering up temptations.

Diabetes support groups: If you are a person with diabetes, then having others around who share similar health experiences and who are trying to adapt their own lives to living with diabetes may be really beneficial. There are many support groups available – whether you find one online or if there is a group in your local area, do take advantage of any support available. There will be lots of tips and advice –from coping with the day-to-day pressures to new recipes that fit your carbohydrate controlled diet. Importantly, this will be information gained through the experience and advice of others who are in a similar situation. Even better, why not start a group approach to the new way of eating and support each other through those early first days?

Family and Friends: It's so good to have the support of your nearest and dearest and whether it is someone to just talk to if you are feeling down, or for when you are tempted to stray from your diet, it can make a huge difference to your success. There will be those who are willing to share your journey and support you throughout and this is significant. Help them by explaining the diet or sharing this book so they know what types of meals and snacks to encourage.

Exercise Buddies: Regular exercise is a vital aspect of changing your life and certainly can become an important part of controlling your diabetes. If you can put in place a dedicated training routine perhaps with a friend – (slowly at first if you haven't exercised much for a while), and to have a progressive plan of action which will enable you to increase the exercise going forward, you will soon start to feel and notice the difference.

Exercise is important because:

- It helps you to control your blood sugar levels
- It helps you to feel good
- It keeps your body healthy and in good shape
- It lowers your blood pressure
- It lowers your heart rate
- It lowers cholesterol levels and triglycerides
- Enables your body to become more insulin sensitive

- Promotes improved blood circulation

CAUTION:
Starting an exercise plan is a positive step but there are times that you should be careful. Make sure you clear any exercise plan through your doctor.

- Check your blood sugar levels prior to starting exercise and after finishing.

- In case of hypoglycemia, carry quick acting carbohydrates that can raise your levels such as: glucose tablets, snacks, or juice.

- Take plenty of water with you to make sure you are well hydrated.

How to Follow the Diet

The Right Quantity of Carbohydrates

When embarking on this new meal plan, it is important that you focus on those all-important carbohydrate percentages and numbers of portions when preparing your food. Each meal should have about 50-60% carbohydrates as we have previously stated and when filling your plate, it should have ½ vegetables (low carbohydrate), ¼ starches, ¼ meats or protein servings. To make it easier, we provide a list of carbohydrates including an insight into vegetables, starches, and proteins. We show how to interpret food labels when shopping, and it is important to pay special attention to those sections as they form the basic foundations of this diet.

Steps to Implement the Diet

When you change an important part of your life, it can be difficult to learn and to incorporate these changes so that they become instinctive. It does mean mastering the basics of carbohydrate counting and learning the essentials so that the relationship between the food you eat, your blood glucose levels and the exercise that you do becomes much clearer. It is like having the pieces of a jigsaw puzzle and slotting all of the information together so that you can see the whole picture. It's about approaching the diet with a sense of clarity and positivity and a good deal of forward planning. The hardest part of making these important changes is learning all about the nutritional aspects rather than just seeing food as nice to eat or something you want and not considering the consequences. Food fuels the body and it makes perfect sense to consider that when you fuel it with low-quality nutrients, it will not perform well. You can use food labels to help you judge the serving sizes and then use that information to determine how much to eat. You can look at the grams of total carbohydrates which include starch, sugar and fiber. Calories are important if you are trying to watch your weight and you need to think about the serving sizes when working out the calorie amounts.

Once you have embraced the concept by figuring out the calories and planning out your day, start considering the foods that you already eat. You may find that more than a few of your old favorites are perfectly acceptable on the diet, or, it may be that you have to tweak them, exchanging fast-burning carbohydrates for a slower and more sustained release option.

1. Prepare some menus utilizing the information within this book.
2. Create a shopping list.
3. Check your food pantry and compare your regular food to those that you should have.

4. Check all of the food labels in the supermarket and choose healthier options.
5. When cooking, think about portion size and quantities using the 50-60% rule.

Many people with diabetes already have a calorie count that they try to follow. **If your doctor or dietitian has recommended a calorie count, use that**. Otherwise, use the information from earlier in the book that talks about how to calculate your caloric level and grams of carbohydrate needed.

HOW TO USE CARBOHYDRATE COUNTING

Learning to use carbohydrate counting on this diet is important. It may sound daunting but it simply means that those foods which contain a similar amount of carbohydrates per serving are then grouped together (like pastas and rice or fruits). You can exchange any of the foods on this list for alternative ones when you are starting to plan your meals. This enables you to stick to the plan but to experiment with ingredients as well using an effective mix and match system. One exchange of carbohydrates equals 15 grams, and if you happen to want another serving of brown rice, you just have to remove/exchange another carbohydrate food that day.

EATING OUT

Once you become familiar with this carbohydrate counting plan, you will find it becomes much easier to enjoy beautiful home-cooked foods that are both tasty and nutritious. Even better, once you get the proportions of carbohydrates right each time you will find that your blood glucose levels fare much better and become more stable. There may be times when you do not wish to cook and choose to go out for a meal instead, but this can be challenging as you will have less control over your carbohydrates as a result.

As time progresses and you become more confident with the diet, you will develop an eye for the correct serving sizes and so, when you are at a restaurant you can look over your food to determine how much you should eat. It helps if you can memorize your meal plan, because this will come in handy when looking at the menu initially. If you have real concerns, call the restaurant in advance and explain your dietary needs or concerns. You will find that most restaurants are quite obliging. Of course this new system is about more than filling your plate with healthy carbohydrates, it's about understanding what certain food types do to your body and about choosing natural wholesome foods. Ask the restaurant any questions if you are unsure. You can also check the website for nutritional information.

Many websites post the nutritional information for their meal and you can select your meal before you even enter the restaurant.

GROCERY SHOPPING TIPS

It can be difficult enough to brave the supermarkets and to avoid all of those cleverly packaged and unhealthy products especially if you feel tired, stressed, or are experiencing a low blood sugar episode. Initially you may feel a bit overwhelmed. Going to the supermarket with a shopping list will help you to avoid being tempted or to add unnecessary items to the cart. It's also a good idea to allow extra time in the supermarket so that you can check those food labels carefully. Success lies in the preparation and many people find that they save money by shopping with a grocery list and meal plan.

When you are at the supermarket, keep in mind that carbohydrates are:

- Starchy foods – cereal, rice, bread

- Fruit and fruit juice

- Yogurt and milk

- Starchy vegetables like potatoes

- Sweets such as cake, sodas, cookies.

Good choices for carbohydrates include: Whole oats, whole grains, pasta, beans and buckwheat, fruits and vegetables including beans, lentils and peas.

Carbohydrate Counting and Label Reading

Carbohydrates in your diet will influence your blood sugars, so planning is essential to control your readings. You will learn how to count carbohydrates (carbs) and read labels so that you are able to plan meals accordingly.

Carbohydrate Counting

It is important that you learn about carb counting. It isn't hard to learn once you know the concept. You will be reading nutritional facts labels to calculate carb units at each meal and snack.

When you look at the serving size, you merely calculate the information provided if you think you would be eating more or less than the example shown. Check out the grams for the total carbohydrate and know that this includes sugar, starch and fiber. Determine your portion size accordingly. Taking this healthy approach one step further, you can also look at the saturated and trans fats per serving and go for the lowest as this will reduce your chance of gaining weight while reducing the risk of heart disease. If you have high blood pressure, reduce the amount of sodium per meal.

There are many different types of sugar that may be shown on the ingredient listing too. For example:

- Glucose
- Sweeteners
- Brown sugar
- Dextrose
- Sucrose
- Fructose
- Galactose
- Raw sugar
- Honey
- Molasses
- Corn sweetener
- Maltose
- High fructose corn syrup
- Sugar
- Sugar alcohols – mannitol, xylitol, sorbitol

You will be a "label reading expert" by the time you are done reading this chapter. Knowing exactly what you put in your mouth is important even when you're not having health issues. Knowing how to read labels will be beneficial now and later.

O.K., let's read our first food label:

Nutrition Facts	Amount/Serving	%DV*	Amount/Serving	%DV*
Serv. size 1 (123g) Servings 4 Calories 230 Fat Cal. 60	Total Fat 6g	10%	Total Carb. 28g	8%
	Sat. Fat 2g	10%	Fiber 0g	0%
	Trans fats 0g		Sugars less than 1g	
* Percent Daily Values (DV) are based on a 2,000 calorie diet.	Cholest. 15mg	4%	Protein 14g	
	Sodium 590mg	25%		
	Vitamin A 4%	Vitamin C 0%	Calcium 20%	Iron 10%

It is important to note what the serving size is. If you don't, you may think a whole packet of food is one serving when it may be three. This label shows that the box contains four servings, and ¼ of the package is a serving. The serving is shown to have 230 calories in it. As you move down the list, you will see the total carbohydrate is 28 grams and there are 0 grams of fiber. That is a very important part of the puzzle and key to pay attention to on the label.

Check out the following chart. By looking at it, you will see that there are two columns. One shows "total carbohydrate grams" and the other is what we call "carbohydrate choices." There are 15 grams of carbohydrate in a carb choice when you are carbohydrate counting. Now, if you are allowed only one carb choice (or 15 grams of carb) for a snack, you wouldn't be able to eat this product.

A way to get some of what you want is if a product had only 25 carbs/2 crackers, you could eat only one cracker and have 12.5 carbohydrates or 1 carb choice.

Total Carbohydrate Grams	Carbohydrate Choices
0-5	0
6-10	½
11-20	1
21-25	1 ½
26-35	2
36-40	2 ½
41-50	3
51-55	3 ½
56-65	4
66-70	4 ½
71-80	5
81-85	5 ½
86-95	6

If you choose this product, you are getting no fiber, but it is high in carbohydrate. However, you may want to choose a smaller serving of a complex carbohydrate such as an apple because you will get more to eat. The apple is low on the glycemic index (discussed later) and more nutritious because it has fiber and will require you to eat more slowly. While you are eating the apple your body has time to register that it is full, and you will likely not eat as much.

Most foods will have the carb count listed on the label but at other times you could need to do a calculation. You calculated the amount of carbohydrates that you needed at a meal and at snacks earlier in this book.

You will see by the chart that the more carbs there are in a food, you will start to use more carb points. How? Let us look at the carb count table: You can see where 11-20 grams of carbohydrates equals one carb choice (or unit). Do you think if you eat 40 grams of carbs of a certain food, you get 2 carb choices? According to the chart, you would get 2 ½. So that ½ carb choice that could've gone to more food is lost on the item you chose. You can't combine all of your carbohydrates for the day or even a meal and apply it to this chart. You will calculate each food as its own carb count.

Let's practice another one:

The following label information is on some nutrition bars. As you can see, the serving size listed here is just one bar. There are twelve servings in the box. Let's take a look at the label and figure out how many carb units are contained.

Nutrition Facts

Serving size: 1 (152g)
Servings Per Recipe   6

Amount Per Serving

Calories 170   Cal. from Fat 50

	% Daily Value*
Total Fat 6g	8%
Saturated Fat 1.5g	8%
Trans Fats 0g	
Cholesterol less than 5mg	2%
Sodium 380mg	15%
Total Carbohydrate 15g	4%
Dietary Fiber 2g	8%
Sugars 2g	
Protein 15g	

Vitamin A	50%	Vitamin C	8%
Calcium	15%	Iron	15%

* Percent Daily Values is based on a 2,000 calorie diet. Your daily values may be higher or lower depending on your calorie needs.

	Calories	2,000	2,500
Total Fat	Less than	65g	80g
Sat Fat	Less than	20g	25g
Cholesterol	Less than	300mg	300mg
Sodium	Less than	2400mg	2400mg
Total Carbohydrate		300g	375g
Dietary Fiber		25g	30g

Calories per gram:
Fat 9   Carbohydrate 4   Protein 4

To count carbohydrates, look at three things:

Serving size

Number of servings per container

Grams of total carbohydrate per serving

Listed in this label are 15 grams of carbohydrates. This lies between 11-20 on the carb unit chart and would count as 1 unit. You are allowed to subtract half the fiber (2 grams) but it wouldn't make much of a significant difference. (And if you ate two, you would get two servings of carbohydrate)

Side note: Sugar alcohols are sometimes added to increase the sweetness but keep the sugar low. Too much of them can cause gastric distress. These are called mannitol or sorbitol in the ingredient listing. You can subtract half their value as well when calculating the carbohydrate count if you find them in foods. They are usually listed under the total carbohydrate section of the label.

This bar counts as 1 carbohydrate serving.

Let's take a look at another potential label.

Nutrition Facts	Amount/Serving	%DV*	Amount/Serving	%DV*
Serv. size 1 (217g)	Total Fat 10g	15%	Total Carb. 13g	4%
Servings 2	Sat. Fat 4.5g	20%	Fiber 3g	10%
Calories 210	Trans fats 0g		Sugars 9g	
Fat Cal. 90	Cholest. 15mg	6%	Protein 16g	
* Percent Daily Values (DV) are	Sodium 220mg	8%		
based on a 2,000 calorie diet.	Vitamin A 15%	Vitamin C 0%	Calcium 8%	Iron 15%

The label above indicates one serving is ½ the recipe (this is for an omelet) and contains 13 grams of carbohydrates. It shows it has 3 grams of dietary fiber. In this example, you would see that 13 grams would convert to 1 carb choices (or units). However, you are allowed to subtract half the dietary fiber from the carbohydrate grams. So 13 grams minus 1.5 grams of dietary fiber brings the total to 11.5 grams. If you look at the carb choice chart again, you will see that this product will still be worth 1 carb choice, but with the 16 gm of protein, it will be a very filling carbohydrate choice.

Let's try another one. Below is a sample food label for a serving of cookies.

Nutrition Facts	Amount/Serving	%DV*	Amount/Serving	%DV*
Serv. size 1 (137g)	Total Fat 16g	25%	Total Carb. 26g	8%
Servings 8	Sat. Fat 7g	35%	Fiber 2g	8%
Calories 310	Trans fats 0g		Sugars 2g	
Fat Cal. 140	Cholest. 205mg	70%	Protein 14g	
* Percent Daily Values (DV) are	Sodium 260mg	10%		
based on a 2,000 calorie diet.	Vitamin A 15%	Vitamin C 25%	Calcium 10%	Iron 10%

The number of carbohydrates is 26 grams, while it contains 2 grams of dietary fiber and 2 grams of sugar. This means you are allowed to subtract half of the dietary fiber. So by taking 26 grams of carbs and subtract 1 grams of fiber, you come up with 26-1=25. These cookies will count as 1 1/2 carb choice.

Be careful with reading the boxes many products are contained in. They may say there are sugar-free but that does not mean they are carbohydrate-free. A sugar-free label means that one serving has less than 0.5 gram of sugar. That is why it is so important to read labels. We need to know how many carbohydrates are in a food before you eat it, not how much sugar is in it. Many labels can be misleading as well. You have to be careful to not assume that a package is a serving size.

Look at this label:

Nutrition Facts	Amount/Serving	%DV*	Amount/Serving	%DV*
Serv. size 1 (471g) Servings 4 Calories 320 Fat Cal. 120	Total Fat 13g	20%	Total Carb. 25g	8%
	Sat. Fat 7g	35%	Fiber less than 1g	2%
	Trans fats 0g		Sugars 2g	
* Percent Daily Values (DV) are based on a 2,000 calorie diet.	Cholest. 80mg	25%	Protein 23g	
	Sodium 450mg	20%		
	Vitamin A 4%	Vitamin C 0%	Calcium 6%	Iron 8%

For this product, if you ate the entire package you would have consumed 6 carbohydrate choices! It contains 4 servings and 25 carbohydrates per serving = 100 gm of carbohydrate and 8 grams of sugar. That would cause a spike in your blood sugar level for sure.

When you're choosing between standard products and their sugar-free counterparts, compare the food labels. If the sugar-free product has noticeably fewer carbohydrates, the sugar-free product might be the better choice. But if there's little difference in carbohydrate grams between the two foods, let taste — or price — be your guide. Remember, a label of "no sugar added" does not mean "no carbohydrates." Although these foods don't contain high-sugar ingredients and no sugar is added during processing or packaging, foods without added sugar may still be high in carbohydrates.

For example, an apple could be labeled "no added sugar" but the natural fructose means that it does contain carbohydrate servings.

Once you get carb counting down, you can start to piece together your meal plan. You will need to know how to count your calories. If your food is packaged, all you need to do is read the label and add the calorie and carbohydrate totals. That will tell you how many carbohydrates you are eating, and allow you to have the flexibility of eating a little of what you want without going overboard.

QUICK STEPS TO GREATER CARBOHYDRATE CONTROL

EASY TO INCORPORATE SUGGESTIONS

Making changes to any diet can be difficult and people approach these changes quite differently. Some people attack the changes with great enthusiasm, relishing each small change to their health and using this for forward momentum. Others need to take smaller steps and to instigate more subtle benefits. Changing your approach to eating carbohydrates will provide many long-term benefits, but it is all about finding the level of carbohydrates that suits your body and it can take a little time to find the right balance.

EAT MORE VEGETABLES

You can eat plenty of low starch and fibrous vegetables on a controlled carbohydrate diet but choose the vegetables carefully. Choose non-starchy alternatives to corn and potatoes and instead use cauliflower, mushrooms, avocado and greens. The following list will give you a good indicator of those vegetables to choose.

Fibrous Vegetables (serving size is ½ cup, approx. 5 gm carbohydrate per serving)

Artichoke/artichoke hearts

Asparagus

Beans (green, wax, Italian)

Bean sprouts

Beets

Broccoli

Brussels sprouts

Carrots

Cauliflower

Celery

Cabbage

Cucumber

Eggplant

Peppers, all varieties

Radishes

Salad greens

Sauerkraut

Spinach

Summer squash

Tomato

Turnips

Water chestnuts

Pea pods

Starchy Vegetables (Each serving is 15 gm carbohydrate)
½ cup corn

1 corn on cob, 6-inch

½ cup peas

1 3oz potato, plain (baked or boiled)

½ cup mashed potatoes

½ cup yam, sweet potato, plain

COUNT AND CONTROL SUGARY OR FRUIT JUICE DRINKS

Many of us turn to sugary drinks throughout the day, preferring them to plain water, but remember that fruit juices still provide carbohydrates so you will need to plan these into your menus. Similarly, if you opt for fruit instead, you may find that you are less hungry, but it still needs to be an allocated part of your allowed carbohydrate for the day.

EMBRACE GOOD FATS

This may seem quite controversial, but fats are important for the body. If you are actually lowering your carbohydrates (because you have always eaten too many) then adding some extra fats is not a bad thing as it can help to fill you up, therefore avoiding hunger pangs. Choose wisely though, by using a good quality olive oil and eating fatty fish, nuts, and seeds. These can help you feel full longer, but they do add calories so use caution when adding to your diet.

FILL UP ON PROTEIN

Because you are aiming for balance on your plate, do make sure that you have regular portions of protein. Approximately 1/4 of your meal should be protein. Protein is usually eaten in the form of chicken, beef, or fish but beans and eggs are also good sources of protein. Just be aware that beans contain carbohydrate as well as protein.

FRESH FOODS

Size proportion is important with a controlled carbohydrate diet, but equally as important is the quality of your food. Enjoy fresh, well-cooked foods that look appealing. Changing your way of eating is not about deprivation; it's about eating well, eating healthy and getting satisfaction from your food while providing your body with all of the necessary nutrients. If you can opt for natural and fresh foods, so much the better.

BROWN VS. WHITE

One great tip when altering your carbohydrate consumption is to select whole-wheat bread instead of white bread and to choose brown rice instead of white rice. These are much healthier options immediately and are a sure-fire way to start making a difference in your diet. Try to avoid white flour and always look to reduce the overall amount of sugar in cooking and meals. You can do this slowly if you have the proverbial sweet tooth, but once you have re-educated those taste buds, you will find that you naturally avoid sweet foods. This isn't about giving up all of your normal food choices, but about making informed choices that will lead to greater health and well-being.

Changes can be difficult at first, but your taste buds will soon adapt, and you will find yourself enjoying your food much more because you know how good it is for your body. Fruits can be an excellent way to get a bit of sweet without too much sugar.

When making the change from white to brown, it is beneficial to gauge the benefits. Brown carbohydrates are those foods or whole grains which are in their natural state e.g., not refined in the way that white carbohydrates are. If we look at whole grains, they still have the kernel intact. The kernel includes the bran, germ, and the endosperm. It contains trace minerals, fiber and B vitamins too.

Whole grains are so much better for your health. Research has indicated that they have been shown to reduce the risk of contracting some cancers and heart disease too. Whole grains also contain antioxidants and phytoestrogens. Whole grains help to control diabetes because they absorb more slowly into the body, and this is a very important aspect of the carbohydrate controlled diet. This is a much better approach than to have the influx of blood sugar from those carbohydrates that are absorbed more quickly. This is why the dramatic highs and lows of blood glucose levels are experienced.

THE GLYCEMIC INDEX OF FOODS

If you have never heard of the Glycemic Index (GI), it is simply the ranking of foods in relation to how quickly they raise your blood glucose levels as compared to regular sugar (100 GI). The lower the glycemic index, the less it affects blood sugar and insulin levels. Imagine it this way – a high GI food is absorbed quickly and raised blood sugar like regular sugar does. A low GI food raises blood sugar more slowly with less of an insulin response from the body.

HIGH GI FOODS (70 +)
White Bread

Bagels

Cornflakes

White Rice

Pasta

Pumpkin

Rice Cakes

Popcorns

Watermelon

Mashed Potato

MEDIUM GI (55-69)
Rye, Pita Bread, Whole Wheat Bread

Couscous

Brown Rice, Basmati Rice, Wild Rice

LOW GI FOODS (55 OR LESS)
100% stone-ground whole wheat or pumpernickel bread

Oatmeal (rolled or steel-cut), oat bran, muesli

Pasta, whole grains, barley, bulgur wheat

Most whole fruits, non-starchy vegetables and carrots

Many beans and nuts

Milk products

When you count carbohydrates you take on a meal-planning technique that works. This is because you keep track of the grams of carbohydrates and set yourself a maximum intake. You consider the target range and then adapt depending on how active you are, and you need to include whether you take medicines as well and how your blood sugars are affected.

The aim of slowing down carbohydrate absorption is beneficial to everyone, simply because there is less stress on the pancreas to release insulin. This can effectively lower the risk of developing diabetes.

Choosing low glycemic index foods helps with your diabetes and overall health. You should try to limit the higher glycemic index foods, because they will increase your blood sugar rapidly and cause your body to release a large amount of insulin – which then creates the cycle where your body stores the additional blood sugar as fat on your body.

CARBOHYDRATE COUNTING PLAN

TOTAL CARBOHYDRATES VS. SUGAR AMOUNT ON LABELS

When planning your carbohydrate intake, it's important to check the food labels of each product that you buy off the shelf, because you may be surprised by the contents within those favorite foods. Labels can be quite misleading. There is so much to check, from counting the calories, to fat grams and sugar content, so where do you start? First, it's important to recognize that all food has a caloric content and they are provided by carbohydrates, proteins and fat. It is probably no surprise to know that fats contain the highest calorie count and is the equivalent to 9 calories for one gram of fat. By comparison, carbohydrates and protein have four calories each per gram. It can help you to consider the food that you eat by reading the labels; they contain the calories per serving and also, the portion size. This list, although complex looking, can point you towards those foods that are much better for you.

While it is important to have some understanding as to how foods affect your body, it is easier to be able to check the food labels and to be able to look at the calorie count, fat levels and carbohydrates as this can provide a quick snapshot of how good the food is going to be for you. Counting calories are important, but do not provide the whole picture. The more you check labels, the easier you will find it to make informed food choices. It's not surprising that there is confusion by the total carbohydrate calculation and grams of sugar but a quick check of the total carbohydrate listing will give you everything that you need. The grams of sugar amount is already included in the total carbohydrate count.

Remember: The total carbohydrate listing contains all the carbohydrate amounts in the food including fiber and sugars.

Your body is finely tuned and needs nutritious foods to be able to perform at an optimal level. Food will affect hormones too, and some hormones serve to release sugar, while other hormones function to build up muscle and some store fat. Reading the food labels provides you with the most accurate way of knowing how many carbohydrates are in any specific foods but sometimes you have to estimate how many carbohydrates are present and you can do this by estimating general foods servings.

There are approximately 15 grams of carbohydrates in the following servings of foods:

Bread
1 slice bread
2 slices low-calorie bread
1 1oz. bread roll
½ hamburger/hot dog bun
½ bagel

½ English muffin

1 2½ -inch biscuit

1 2-inch cube cornbread

½ 6-inch pita

1 6-inch tortilla

2 6-inch taco shells

1 4½ -inch waffle

1 slice French toast

1 cup croutons

1/3 cup bread stuffing

1/4 inch thick pancake

Crackers and Snacks

15-20 tortilla or potato chips

24 oyster crackers

8 animal crackers

¾ oz pretzels

3 cups ready popcorn

2 4-inch rice cakes

½ cup chow mein noodles

3 cheese or peanut butter crackers

Cereals and Grains

½ cereal bar

½ unfrosted Poptart

¾ cup unsweetened cereal

½ cup sugar-frosted cereal

½ cup bran cereal

1 ½ cup puffed cereal

½ cup Shredded Wheat®

½ cup oats (cooked)

1/3 cup couscous (cooked)

3 Tbsp cornmeal (dry)

3 Tbsp wheat germ

½ cup pasta (cooked)

1/3 cup rice (white or brown) (cooked)

½ cup rice milk

3 Tbsp dry flour

Starchy Vegetables
½ cup corn

1 6 – inch corn on cob

½ cup peas

1 3oz baked or boiled potato, plain

½ cup mashed potatoes

½ cup yam, sweet potato, plain

1 cup squash, winter (acorn, butternut)

1 ½ cup vegetable juice

1/3 – 1/2 cup tomato or spaghetti sauce

Milk and Yogurt
1 cup (8 oz) skim milk

¾ cup (6 oz) plain, low-fat yogurt

½ cup evaporated milk

1/3 cup non-fat dry milk

Fruit

½ cup canned fruit (unsweetened and in its own juice)

1 small banana (approximately 4 inches)

1 small apple or orange

15 small grapes

1¼ cup strawberries, whole

1¼ cup watermelon (cubed)

1 cup cantaloupe, honeydew, papaya (cubed)

2 tbsp raisins

¼ cup dried fruit

½ cup juice (apple, grapefruit, orange pineapple)

1/3 cup juice (grape, cranberry, prune, blends)

Fibrous Vegetables

Each item listed contains **about 5 grams of carbohydrate per serving**. A serving is counted as ½ cup of cooked vegetables or 1 cup of raw vegetables.

Artichoke/artichoke hearts

Asparagus

Beans (green, wax, Italian)

Bean sprouts

Beets

Broccoli

Brussels sprouts

Cabbage

Carrots

Cauliflower

Protein/Fat (0 grams carbohydrate)

Each item listed is considered a protein and/or fat, unless you add carbohydrate to it.

Beef

Poultry

Fish

Seafood

Pork

Veal

Luncheon/deli meats

Eggs

Cheese

Nuts

Olive Oil

It is much easier when you can gauge the carbohydrate content by looking at the individual food labels. Not only can you see easily how many carbohydrates are present, you can also determine how much of it you should eat. The serving size is important.

Although this book concentrates on counting those all-important carbs, just remember that you must have fats and proteins to ensure that your meal is balanced. All nutrients are important.

Learning your list of carbohydrates is important because it may seem to the uninformed eye that carbohydrates are not included but, they can come from other foods for example – flour. Read the label for the total carbohydrate amount and not the sugar amount only.

Fats and Oils

Awareness of the good and bad fats makes a great start for your health. Know which ones to avoid, but to still include the good fats so that you are eating a healthy diet. Fats are either saturated or unsaturated and it is wise to choose unsaturated fats. Depending on your health needs, do be aware that all fats can and do help you to put on weight because they are concentrated sources of calories.

Saturated fats and trans fats are found in animal products, butter, cheese, whole milk, cream, pastries, pies, prepared desserts, and biscuits. They are linked with obesity and high cholesterol levels. They are solid at room temperature – like butter. You should try to limit your intake of these types of fats.

Unsaturated fats include: monounsaturated and polyunsaturated. Omega -9 (also called Oleic acid) is the main monounsaturated fats and is found in seeds, avocados, olive oil, ground nut oil, sunflower oil, avocados, nuts.

Polyunsaturated fats include: Omega -3s and Omega-6s. Fatty acids within these two groups are called alpha-linolenic acid and linoleic acid. They are often deemed essential fatty acids. This is because the human body is unable to create them directly due to the lack of enzymes so it is important to obtain them from the diet. As long as you eat a variety of foods and ingest more than 10 gm of fat per day, you will receive the essential fatty acids you need in your diet.

If you are confused by all of the different fats and have no idea which ones to incorporate and those that you should avoid, the good news is that not all fats are bad. Fats to avoid are trans fats and saturated fats as these are problematic for clogging up the arteries and for putting on weight. Good fats include the polyunsaturated fats, monounsaturated fats, and omega 3s and they can help with heart health and lowering cholesterol. Olive oil and canola oil are the best oils to cook with, although sunflower oil contains beneficial fats as well.

When you consider fat consumption in your diet, it makes sense to reduce the overall quantity of fats within your food but in particular, to reduce substantially the amount of fats that are part of the 'bad fat' list. Surprisingly, the good fats can actually help with mood management, weight control and can even help to lessen feelings of fatigue.

HYDROGENATED OILS

You may well have heard about the perils of hydrogenated oil but what actually is it and why is it so bad? They are quite healthy when in their natural state but the actual process and manufacturing turn them into poisons. It may sound dramatic but actually, this is really the case. The oils – from palm, soybean, and coconut oil are heated to up to one thousand degrees. A catalyst is injected into the oil, this is nickel, aluminum or platinum and this starts to change the molecular structure so it becomes semi-solid or solid oil turning into partially or fully hydrogenated oils. Essentially, the oils are no longer natural and are unhealthy when consumed.

It is important that you stay away from hydrogenated oils where possible, although this can be typically hard to do because it is in so much of what we eat. The trick is to eat your food as close to its natural state and raw where possible. Essentially this means eating more fruits and vegetables and fresh meat from local sources when available. Hydrogenated oils are within packaged and processed foods so if you can avoid buying food that is highly processed directly off the shelf, then you will be eating much healthier anyway. Hydrogenated oils serve to extend the shelf-life of products and are known to be hard on your arteries.

GOOD FATS

Monounsaturated Fats

Olive oil

Canola oil

Sunflower oil

Peanut oil

Sesame oil

Avocados

Nuts (almonds, peanuts, macadamia nuts, hazelnuts, pecans, cashews)

Peanut butter

Olives

Polyunsaturated Fats

Soybean oil

Corn oil

Safflower oil

Walnuts

Sunflower, sesame, and pumpkin seeds

Flaxseed

Fatty fish (salmon, tuna, mackerel, herring, trout, sardines)

Soymilk

Tofu

BAD FATS

Saturated Fats

High-fat cuts of meat (lamb, pork and beef) – trim before cooking

Chicken with the skin – remove the skin before cooking

Whole-fat dairy products (milk and cream)

Butter

Cheese

Ice cream

Palm and coconut oil

Lard

Trans Fats and Hydrogenated Oils
Cookies, biscuits, commercially baked pastries, doughnuts, muffins, cakes,

Pizza dough

Stick margarine

Vegetable shortening

Fried foods (French fries, fried chicken, chicken nuggets, breaded fish)

Candy bars

It's important that when you undertake the carbohydrate controlled diet that you re-think your understanding of food and consider packaged foods a "no-go" area while natural and unprocessed foods as the best you can have. This means that anytime you do have to buy any packaged food, you need to read the labels carefully to make certain the product does not contain hydrogenated oils. Don't be fooled by marketing and fancy labeling either. The product may have the word organic written across it, but that does not necessarily mean that it is really healthy. If you want healthy food, these items need to have all of their natural vitamins, minerals, and enzymes. This means eating foods that are as near to their natural and unprocessed state as possible and that ideally you have researched and cooked for yourself.

Hydrogenated oils are an ingredient that really should be avoided, but it's not just found in the supermarkets but when you eat out too. Many restaurants use hydrogenated oils as well, so limit those meals out especially when you first start trying to embark on the diet. It has to become second nature.

THE FIRST WEEK

THE PATH TO SUCCESS

The first week can be understandably difficult when you are
making such considerable changes to your diet. Don't despair
though. It's all about helping your body to adjust to what might
be extensive changes depending on what your diet was like
before. It's not easy to predict exactly how you will feel during
the first week. If you were on a high carbohydrate diet
previously then you may feel less energetic in the first few days
as your body adjusts. When your body has fewer carbohydrates,
it has to use fat instead and convert that to energy, which is a
good process for your body to do. But this is not about going
onto a low carbohydrate diet, but maintaining consistency with
portion sizes and eating a balanced amount of carbohydrate at
each meal.

In the first three days, you may find that you experience some
withdrawal symptoms. You are changing the quantities and are
eating less by comparison, and it can feel as if you are missing
out. If you do find yourself struggling and longing for a big plate
of pasta, hold out, because you will soon start to feel better. Eat
some additional fibrous vegetables to hold you over. You are
changing old habits and this does not always come easy. In fact,
your mind will often hold on to the old ways of living so you
have a silent battle when trying to adopt healthier ways to live.

So it is more than the actual dietary changes that you will find hard to cope with.

PLAN DELICIOUS FOOD TO KEEP YOU ON THE STRAIGHT AND NARROW

Planning healthy but tasty foods to eat can help you to stay focused and to not veer off your healthy eating plan. Once you start to understand all of the important aspects of this regime, then it will be much easier to plan in some tasty treats without causing a problem to the overall diet. Make sure you do not start getting hungry. If you have the right proportion of carbs and are eating consistently, then this should not happen but, if you do start feeling hungry, go for a no-carb option which typically is meat, fish and some dairy products. Many vegetables make good snacks for between meals since they are low in carbohydrate but filling.

GROCERY SHOPPING FOR THE FIRST TIME

Going shopping for the first time when starting a carbohydrate controlled diet, can be very daunting especially if you are used to buy certain food types and may have not indulged in writing out a nutritious diet plan for some time. The important thing here to consider is the recipes that you are likely to have for the first time and what carbohydrates are included. Food such as: brown rice, whole-wheat bread, beans, berries, whole grain pastas, and leafy-green vegetables are good to add to the shopping cart as they are a good source of carbohydrates, but also have an abundance of nutrients and fiber.

DRINK WATER
Regardless of any new health changes, it is important to keep drinking plenty of fresh water as this will also help you to think and feel with greater clarity, it helps with your concentration levels and will make you look more energized. Check the labels of water as some will have had extra sugars added to them and these could very quickly raise your blood sugar quickly. Stick to plain water – add a squirt of lemon if you need some flavor.

REWARD YOURSELF
It's good to reward yourself when you have made such positive changes to your life. In fact, by the end of the first week you should really start to feel the benefits of eating healthier. You will have a greater understanding of how the dietary changes work and a heightened sense of awareness and increased sense of energy. It can really help at the start of the week to plan a treat for the end of that first week so that you have something to aim for and can celebrate. The treat can be anything healthy, an evening out at the theatre, a moonlit walk along the beach, or anything that really makes you feel good.

Correcting Mistakes

If you are new to calculating your carbohydrates and trying to move away from an unhealthy diet, there is no doubt you will make a mistake or two. If you have diabetes, then it is of course even more important to monitor your menus and to carefully select the food types so that you give yourself the best opportunity for maintaining glucose levels in your blood. But if you do make mistakes, don't despair, learn from them and then resolve to not make the same mistake again.

There is a lot to comprehend when it comes to food and what is healthy and what is not and unfortunately, this is because; we muddy the waters for ourselves. Manufacturers add all sorts of unhealthy chemicals into the process or tamper with the basic structures of our foods and then we wonder why we are not so healthy. The best way to live is as naturally as possible. It's a learning curve, but, an important one.

Giving Up Too Easily

You will hear lots of information about different types of diets and the importance of restricting carbs, but do remember that for a healthy diet, while you need to be carb aware, you are not trying to reduce the amount of carbs that you eat to nothing. You are trying to consider food portions and to aim for quality foods that tantalize the taste buds but leave you feeling nourished for a longer period of time. When you change your diet, there can naturally be a slump when things start to go wrong or it becomes hard work. Just remember that in the first few days or weeks, you will have to consider every little thing, but once you have accrued this knowledge, you will find it much easier going forward.

EATING VEGETABLES

The most important thing to consider with your carbohydrate controlled diet is to consider that 50-60% of your meal (each meal) should contain carbohydrates and preferably the good carbs e.g., unprocessed. Many people feel that they have to reduce their portions of vegetables but this is not the case, they simply need to think about the portion sizes. So yes, you can have fruits and vegetables because it is all about balancing the diet and maintaining energy levels. When dishing up your plate, consider the types of carbohydrates you are eating and this awareness will help to ensure you stick to the regime more readily.

Vegetables have some carbohydrates and you do need to be aware of this when you are considering your menus for the week. You also have to consider the type of carbohydrates.

Vegetables are divided into starchy and non-starchy types and knowledge of the different types alone with the category in which they are placed is important. Starchy vegetables contain more carbohydrates than non-starchy.

When counting carbohydrates, assume that 15 grams of carbohydrates is equal to one serving. It's a complex affair to calculate the amount of carbohydrates needed based on your calorie requirement, which can also help to maintain weight. If you were planning a 1500 calories a day diet you would need 12-13 servings of carbohydrates a day.

Let's do the math:

1500 calories X 50% Carbohydrate – 750 calories from carbohydrate

750 calories / 4 calories per gram of carbohydrate = 187.5 gm of carbohydrate per day

187.5 gm carbohydrate / 15 gm per serving = 12.5 servings per day of carbohydrate

Fortunately, food labels do reveal serving sizes and the grams of carbohydrates to make it easier.

Starchy Vegetables (1/2 cup cooked) (15 gm carbohydrate per serving)
Peas

Potatoes

Winter squash

Yams

Butternut squash

Sweet potatoes

Parsnips

Non-Starchy Vegetables (1/2 cup cooked or 1 cup raw) (5 gm carbohydrate per serving)

Cauliflower

Cabbage

Peppers

Cucumbers

Greens

Carrots

Broccoli

Brussels sprouts

Bean sprouts

Beetroot

Asparagus

Artichoke

Celery

Eggplant

Leeks

Mushrooms

Radishes

Okra

Turnips

Water chestnuts

Spinach

Watercress

Chicory

Lettuce

Endive

All vegetables are an excellent source of nutrition but if you have been diagnosed with type 2 diabetes then you will need to limit the number of starchy vegetables. These are not bad vegetables as they do have health benefits and serve to fill you up. Starchy foods should not be eaten with abandon.

FIBER

People worry about not eating enough fiber but if you are eating plenty of fruit and vegetables on your carbohydrate controlled diet, then don't worry, you will be eating quite a bit of natural fiber this way. Fiber after all, is simply the part of the plant that we are unable to digest and so it passes through the digestive system without being broken down or absorbed. Most people think about fiber being useful for the prevention of constipation. It has other benefits too, including lowering the impact of starches and sugars on blood glucose. It is also considered beneficial for lowering the risk of heart disease.

FOOD RUTS

When you start out on any diet, whether it is to specifically lose weight or, like this one, to help promote energy levels while maintaining regular glucose levels, you have to be careful to not get into a rut. This is because once you find food combinations that you like and are confident with, it's easy to stop being adventurous and very easy to use the same recipes over and over. Try to keep coming up with alternatives so that you do not get bored with your menus. Keep checking labels and trying new fruits and vegetables to improve the variety in your diet.

The delicate balance between your "safe" meals – foods and combinations you know are good for you – and boredom should be reviewed. If you are happy with your meals and find them easy to stick to – don't change as long as they are working.

Losing Momentum

You start to feel better. Your health has improved substantially, your mood is stable as are your blood sugar levels, you feel more energized and then suddenly, old habits start to creep back into your diet. You have some extra toast, you skip meals or you reach out for some bad foods – just this once but before you know it, you have slipped back into your old routine. Don't fall into this common trap, be aware that sometimes you will slip off the straight and narrow but remember to get back on track and focus. Your health is at stake.

RECIPES

So you have read the book and should have a fairly good idea of the concept of counting those carbohydrates. Don't worry if you have to go back over and recap any of the information within these pages, it's only natural that you may have questions and no doubt will make some mistakes as you learn. Use this book as a point of reference going forward and enjoy experimenting with food.

As much as this dietary plan is about portion size –it's about counting carbohydrates and working out the right amount of carbohydrates per day in relation to an exercise plan that works for you. It's a fine balance and you will get better with time and be able to manage how you eat and improve your energy. Check your blood sugar levels regularly, and you will know if you are eating too many carbohydrates or not enough. When you can balance your carbohydrate intake, you will find that your blood sugar levels remain constant.

The good news is that anyone can learn the basics of this dietary plan; it just takes a little practice. You need to understand which foods are carbohydrates and of course how many carbs are contained within them. When you buy food at your local supermarket, the nutritional values will all be printed on the back and this will also show you the 'total carbohydrates' within a single serving. If you are buying packaged foods, then the serving size information might be a little misleading (probably sometimes a little smaller than you thought), and you may have to calculate the serving as required by you. Also check the labels to determine if a food is sugar-free. **Note that sugar-free does not mean carbohydrate free.**

You will soon get used to looking at food labels but if you are creating recipes or following recipes, then it will be easier for you to look up the carbohydrate values for individual ingredients. If we use a sandwich as an example, you would have to count the carbs for both slices of bread and then check the carb value of any sandwich filling.

There are carbohydrate counters available which will make life a whole lot simpler and here is a link to a website where you can very quickly check the carb quantities for your meals. – http://www.lillydiabetes.com/Pages/carbohydrate-counter.aspx

RECIPES:

Food does not need to be dull on this diet. You can be as creative as you like as long as you follow the rules. Consider ingredients and serving sizes when preparing and adjust accordingly.

BREAKFASTS

Egg and Avocado

1 poached egg

1/2 avocado – peeled and sliced

Mushrooms (1/4 cup boiled)

2 slices of whole-wheat bread

1 tsp butter

1 cup of coffee or tea

Place poached egg, mushrooms and avocado in a stack on one lightly buttered slice of bread and then finish with the second slice of bread.

Nutrition Facts	Amount/Serving	%DV*	Amount/Serving	%DV*
Serv. size 1 (258g) Servings 1 **Calories** 440 Fat Cal. 230	**Total Fat** 26g	**40%**	**Total Carb.** 38g	**15%**
	Sat. Fat 7g	**35%**	Fiber 12g	**45%**
	Trans fats 0g		Sugars 5g	
	Cholest. 220mg	**70%**	**Protein** 17g	
* Percent Daily Values (DV) are based on a 2,000 calorie diet.	**Sodium** 610mg	**25%**		
	Vitamin A 4%	Vitamin C 15%	Calcium 15%	Iron 20%

Fruit Breakfast

1 cup of fresh blackberries

1 cup of fresh strawberries

1 cup of canned peaches (halves)

1 tsp honey

Water

Place required amount of fruit in a bowl and drizzle with a little honey.

Water to drink afterwards.

Nutrition Facts	Amount/Serving	%DV*	Amount/Serving	%DV*
Serv. size 1 (416g) Servings 1 **Calories** 200 **Fat Cal.** 10	**Total Fat** 1.5g	**2%**	**Total Carb.** 49g	**15%**
	Sat. Fat 0g	**0%**	Fiber 11g	**45%**
	Trans fats 0g		Sugars 32g	
* Percent Daily Values (DV) are based on a 2,000 calorie diet.	**Cholest.** 0mg	**0%**	**Protein** 4g	
	Sodium 10mg	**0%**		
	Vitamin A 10%	Vitamin C 200%	Calcium 8%	Iron 10%

Bagel Delight

1 whole wheat bagel (3 ounces)

1/2 small banana

1 tsp honey

Cup of coffee or tea.

Mash the banana and add to the top of the bagel. Drizzle a little honey on the top.

Nutrition Facts	Amount/Serving	%DV*	Amount/Serving	%DV*
Serv. size 1 (155g) Servings 1 **Calories** 310 **Fat Cal.** 15	**Total Fat** 1.5g	**4%**	**Total Carb.** 65g	**20%**
	Sat. Fat 0g	**0%**	Fiber 5g	**20%**
	Trans fats 0g		Sugars 18g	
	Cholest. 0mg	**0%**	**Protein** 11g	
* Percent Daily Values (DV) are based on a 2,000 calorie diet.	**Sodium** 430mg	**20%**		
	Vitamin A 0%	Vitamin C 8%	Calcium 2%	Iron 15%

Simple Spirals

2 ounces of whole wheat pasta spirals

½ cup of jarred pasta sauce

Cup of sugar free iced tea

Boil ½ cup of pasta noodles until softened, about 8 minutes. Add pasta sauce and stir.

Nutrition Facts	Amount/Serving	%DV*	Amount/Serving	%DV*
Serv. size 1 (189g)	Total Fat 3g	4%	Total Carb. 53g	20%
Servings 1	Sat. Fat 0g	2%	Fiber 2g	10%
Calories 260	Trans fats 0g		Sugars 7g	
Fat Cal. 25	Cholest. less than 5mg	1%	Protein 10g	
* Percent Daily Values (DV) are	Sodium 560mg	25%		
based on a 2,000 calorie diet.	Vitamin A 15%	Vitamin C 4%	Calcium 6%	Iron 15%

Mustard Chicken

4 ounces boneless, skinless chicken breast

2 tablespoons mustard with ½ cup of chicken broth

¼ cup sliced onions

¼ cup rice, uncooked

Mix together the broth and mustard. In a medium saucepan, poor broth over chicken and cook slowly. About five minutes on each side.   Add chopped mushrooms and chopped onions – then continue another 10 minutes.

Boil the rice and serve.

Nutrition Facts	Amount/Serving	%DV*	Amount/Serving	%DV*
Serv. size 1 (323g) Servings 1 **Calories** 360 Fat Cal. 40	**Total Fat** 4.5g	**8%**	**Total Carb.** 44g	**15%**
	Sat. Fat 1g	**4%**	Fiber less than 1g	**6%**
	Trans fats 0g		Sugars 2g	
* Percent Daily Values (DV) are based on a 2,000 calorie diet.	**Cholest.** 75mg	**25%**	**Protein** 32g	
	Sodium 870mg	**35%**		
	Vitamin A 0%	Vitamin C 4%	Calcium 4%	Iron 6%

Zucchini Fritters

1 medium zucchini – diced

1 Tbsp olive oil

1 large beaten egg

1/3 cup skim milk

2 tablespoons corn

½ cup self-rising flour

Black pepper to taste

¼ tsp Oregano

Lettuce leaves

Whisk the egg, milk, zucchini, and corn. Then add pepper, mixed herbs, and stir in the flour. Heat the oil in a frying pan. Spoon small dollops of the zucchini mixture into the oil and fry slowly. Turn them and place on a paper towel to drain any excess oil. Prepare lettuce leaves, place the fritters on top, and serve.

Nutrition Facts	Amount/Serving	%DV*	Amount/Serving	%DV*
Serv. size 1 (461g) Servings 1	Total Fat 20g	30%	Total Carb. 65g	20%
Calories 510	Sat. Fat 4g	20%	Fiber 5g	20%
Fat Cal. 180	Trans fats 0g		Sugars 10g	
	Cholest. 190mg	60%	Protein 19g	
* Percent Daily Values (DV) are based on a 2,000 calorie diet.	Sodium 870mg	35%		
	Vitamin A 20%	Vitamin C 60%	Calcium 40%	Iron 30%

Herbed Salmon and Vegetables

5 oz fillet of salmon

1 teaspoon dry Tarragon

1 teaspoon crushed coriander seeds

1 tablespoon freshly squeezed lemon juice

1 teaspoon butter

1 cup cauliflower

1 cup broccoli

1 small potato (baked)

½ cup picante sauce

Bake a medium sized potato in the oven for 50 minutes or in the microwave for 7 minutes. Prepare cauliflower and broccoli. Marinate the fish in butter, herbs and lemon juice for four minutes altogether, then bake salmon in oven for 20 minutes or until done. When ready, serve.

Nutrition Facts	Amount/Serving	%DV*	Amount/Serving	%DV*
Serv. size 1 (588g) Servings 1	Total Fat 24g	35%	Total Carb. 47g	15%
Calories 540	Sat. Fat 7g	35%	Fiber 10g	40%
Fat Cal. 210	Trans fats 0g		Sugars 11g	
	Cholest. 90mg	30%	Protein 37g	
* Percent Daily Values (DV) are based on a 2,000 calorie diet.	Sodium 660mg	30%		
	Vitamin A 20%	Vitamin C 290%	Calcium 10%	Iron 20%

Garlic Chicken and Potato Wedges

4 ounces chicken breast fillet

1 tablespoon butter

1 small potato – chopped into wedges

1 teaspoon dried rosemary

Garlic to taste

Lettuce leaves chopped

Marinate the chicken fillet in garlic butter until cooked.

Chop one potato into chunky wedges – drizzle with a little olive oil and sprinkle with dried rosemary to taste. Add a little chopped fresh garlic into the oven dish and cook for 30-40 minutes until done.

Prepare lettuce leaves and place the chicken fillet on the bed of leaves with a side portion of potato wedges.

Nutrition Facts	Amount/Serving	%DV*	Amount/Serving	%DV*
Serv. size 1 (251g) Servings 1	Total Fat 15g	25%	Total Carb. 18g	6%
Calories 320	Sat. Fat 8g	40%	Fiber 3g	15%
Fat Cal. 130	Trans fats 0g		Sugars 2g	
	Cholest. 105mg	35%	Protein 29g	
* Percent Daily Values (DV) are based on a 2,000 calorie diet.	Sodium 85mg	4%		
	Vitamin A 8%	Vitamin C 20%	Calcium 4%	Iron 6%

Chicken and Asparagus Rice

1/2 cup chicken broth

1 tablespoon olive oil

1 tsp chopped garlic

4 ounces boneless chicken breasts

1 chopped onion

1/4 cup brown rice

4 ounces white wine

1 cup asparagus

Pinch dried basil

Ground pepper

1 tablespoon parmesan cheese

Heat olive oil in a sauce pan. Stir in chopped garlic – cook for 20 seconds. Add diced chicken and cook until chicken is cooked. Place chicken to one side.

In the same saucepan, add chopped onions and cook until softened. Stir in brown rice. Cook until the rice becomes opaque in color. Add the asparagus and stir in the wine. When wine has evaporated, reduce the heat and then stir in ½ cup chicken broth. Continue to cook and stir for up to 10 minutes until the liquid has absorbed. Season. Pour ½ cup water and repeat.

Finally season, stir in the cheese with the chicken and serve hot.

Nutrition Facts	Amount/Serving	%DV*	Amount/Serving	%DV*
Serv. size 1 (647g)	Total Fat 21g	30%	Total Carb. 57g	20%
Servings 1	Sat. Fat 4.5g	20%	Fiber 6g	25%
Calories 680	Trans fats 0g		Sugars 7g	
Fat Cal. 190	Cholest. 100mg	35%	Protein 47g	
* Percent Daily Values (DV) are	Sodium 650mg	25%		
based on a 2,000 calorie diet.	Vitamin A 25%	Vitamin C 80%	Calcium 15%	Iron 20%

Summary and Next Steps

It's never easy to absorb the complete science behind a change in diet but these recipes form a great starting point and indicate the types of menus that can be slotted together easily. Remember that carbohydrates provide you with energy so make the most of this additional energy and embark on a gentle fitness plan. This will ensure that you do not experience weight-gain if you are increasing your carbohydrate intake, but will actually find that you tone up and lose weight once you have the right balance. Any type of diet should be about a whole mind and body approach, and if you can control your diabetes, increase your energy, and take better care of your nutritional needs, it makes sense to incorporate these changes now.

Don't just put this book down, do a few things to get you started on the right track!

1. Calculate your calories using the worksheet on the next few pages. It provides several options for how to figure out what your calorie level is. If you need more help, re-read pages: 27 – 29

2. Make an eating pattern based on your calorie level. Divide the day up into 3 to 4 meals and snacks. Figure out how many carbohydrates you can have at a meal.

3. Make a meal plan for your next week – using some of these recipes or ones that you already have. Review the carbohydrate amounts in your recipes. Remember to add a lot of fresh vegetables to your meals so you are feeling full.

4. Follow the meal pattern and note where you get hungry or tired. This could signal the need for an adjustment.

5. Add exercise a little at a time – don't overdo it.

6. Good luck! Send me a note at contact@healthydietmenusforyou.com if you have any questions or problems.

WORKSHEETS:

Quick Method Based on Bodyweight

Multiply your current bodyweight in pounds times the multiplier number that best fits your situation.

To Lose Weight: Multiply your weight in pounds:
_____ X 12 =
_____ calories needed
[for example if you weigh 160 pounds X 12 = 1960 calories per day]
You may want to subtract an additional 250 – 500 calories per day if you are not losing weight on this amount of calories.

To Maintain Your Weight: your weight in pounds:
_____ X 15 =
_____ calories needed
[for example if you weigh 160 pounds X 15 = 2400 calories per day]

To Gain Weight: your weight in pounds:
_____ X 18 =
_____ calories needed
[for example if you weigh 160 pounds X 18 = 2880 calories per day]
These equations are quick estimations, and may not be the most accurate method. If you are extremely active, you may require more calories, and if you are inactive or have a large amount of body fat, you may require less calories. It's a good starting point.

Equations Based On Basal Metabolic Rate

English BMR Formula

Women: BMR = 655 + (4.35 x weight in pounds) + (4.7 x height in inches) - (4.7 x age in years)

Men: BMR = 66 + (6.23 x weight in pounds) + (12.7 x height in inches) - (6.8 x age in year)

Metric BMR Formula

Women: BMR = 655 + (9.6 x weight in kilos) + (1.8 x height in cm) - (4.7 x age in years)

Men: BMR = 66 + (13.7 x weight in kilos) + (5 x height in cm) - (6.8 x age in years)

Women: 1. 4.35 X _____ (weight in pounds) = _____(a)

Women: 2. 4.7 X _____ (height in inches) = _____(b)

Women: 3. 4.7 X _____ (age in years) = _____(c)

Equation: 655 + _____(a) + _____(b) - _____(c)

Men: 1. 6.23 X _____ (weight in pounds) = _____(a)

Men: 2. 12.7 X _____ (height in inches) = _____(b)

Men: 3. 6.8 X _____ (age in years) = _____(c)

Equation: 66 + _____(a) _____ (b)- _____(c)

Now take your basal metabolic rate and multiply it by an activity factor:

Sedentary = BMR X 1.2 (little or no exercise, desk job)

Lightly Active = BMR X 1.375 (light exercise, sports 1-3 days per week)

Moderately Active = BMR X 1.55 (moderate exercise, 3-5 days per week)

Very Active = BMR X 1.725 (hard exercise, 6-7 days per week)

For example, a woman who weighs 160 pounds, is 62 inches tall, 40 years old and is sedentary
in her activity level would calculate like this:

Women: 1. 4.35 X _160_ = 696(a)

2. 4.7 X __62___ = 291 (b)

3. 4.7 X __40_ = 188 (c)

Equation: 655 + 696 + 291 - 188 = 1454

Sedentary = BMR X 1.2 = 1454 X 1.2 = 1745 calories needed per day

Other Titles By Mathea Ford:

Mathea Ford, Author Page (all books):

http://www.amazon.com/Mathea-Ford/e/B008E1E7IS/

The Kidney Friendly Diet Cookbook

http://www.amazon.com/Kidney-Friendly-Diet-Cookbook-PreDialysis-ebook/dp/B00BC7BGPI/

Create Your Own Kidney Diet Plan

http://www.amazon.com/Create-Your-Kidney-Diet-Plan-ebook/dp/B009PSN3R0/

Living with Chronic Kidney Disease - Pre-Dialysis

http://www.amazon.com/Living-Chronic-Kidney-Disease-Pre-Dialysis-ebook/dp/B008D8RSAQ/

Eating a Pre-Dialysis Kidney Diet - Calories, Carbohydrates, Fat & Protein, Secrets To Avoid Dialysis

http://www.amazon.com/Eating-Pre-Dialysis-Kidney-Diet-Carbohydrates-ebook/dp/B00DU2JCHM/

Eating a Pre-Dialysis Kidney Diet - Sodium, Potassium, Phosphorus and Fluids, A Kidney Disease Solution

http://www.amazon.com/Eating-Pre-Dialysis-Kidney-Diet-Phosphorus-ebook/dp/B00E2U8VMS/

Eating Out On a Kidney Diet: Pre-dialysis and Diabetes: Ways To Enjoy Your Favorite Foods

http://www.amazon.com/Eating-Out-Kidney-Diet-Pre-dialysis/dp/0615928781/

Kidney Disease: Common Labs and Medical Terminology: The Patient's Perspective

http://www.amazon.com/Kidney-Disease-Terminology-Perspective-Pre-Dialysis/dp/0615931804/

Dialysis: Treatment Options for the Progression to End Stage Renal Disease

http://www.amazon.com/Dialysis-Treatment-Options-Progression-Disease/dp/0615932258/

Mindful Eating For A Pre-Dialysis Kidney Diet: Healthy Attitudes Toward Food and Life

http://www.amazon.com/Mindful-Eating-Pre-Dialysis-Kidney-Diet/dp/0615933475/

The Emotional Challenges Of Coping with Chronic Kidney Disease

http://www.amazon.com/Emotional-Challenges-Chronic-Disease-Dialysis-ebook/dp/B00H6SYQG8/

Heart Healthy Living with Kidney Disease: Lowering Blood Pressure

http://www.amazon.com/Heart-Healthy-Living-Kidney-Disease/dp/0615936059/

Exercising with Chronic Kidney Disease: Solutions To An Active Lifestyle

http://www.amazon.com/Exercising-Chronic-Kidney-Disease-Solutions/dp/0615936342/

Sign up for our email list to learn of new titles right away!

http://www.healthydietmenusforyou.com

www.ingramcontent.com/pod-product-compliance
Lightning Source LLC
Chambersburg PA
CBHW070940210326
41520CB00021B/6988